How Our Family Survived

10 Ways to Holistically Manage Childhood Cancer...and Fostering!

By Mandy Lee

www.FosteringNutrition.com

Lived and written by
Mandy Lee, Mom, B.S., NTP, Founder of Fostering
Nutrition(.com)
©2013 Blume and Grow Healthy LLC

ISBN: 1505216710
ISBN-13: 978-1505216714

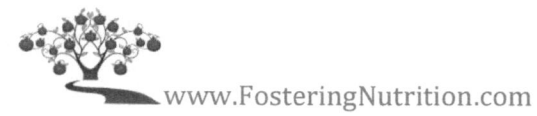

www.FosteringNutrition.com

Reviews

This eBook is a must-read. So many "a-ha!" moments that are sure to make you smile, cry and reflect on the very essence of your being. Mandy Lee shows how to be healthy in mind, body, and spirit and challenges all of us to take on a little more of life. -Krista Butler, B.A., M.Sc., NTP, www.BeFoodSavvy.com

Inspirational on all levels. Living healthy is truly a life-long goal and Mandy Lee shows how important it is to share what we have been given and to help out others. -Dr. Joe Christiano, author and speaker of different body and blood types, author of best seller, Bloodtypes, Bodytypes and You and The Answer is in YOUR Bloodtype.

This is the inspiring book that shows you how to overcome the challenges of illness in families today. On a day-to-day basis, we all face choices in how to eat healthy. If this family can find a way, certainly anyone can! -Kristin Clough Canty, "Adventures in Food, Farm, and Film" blog, and director of the documentary Farmageddon, The Unseen War on American Family Farms.

Many thanks to Kristen Ethridge, author of Saving Gracie, Books by Kristen Ethridge, for taking time to edit my errors and share her writing expertise.

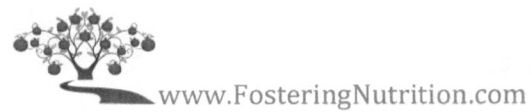 www.FosteringNutrition.com

In Memory of

Our inspiration

**Dak, our foster-to-adopt son

2006 - 2010

With great appreciation

*To my blessed family: Thank you for
understanding why Mommy couldn't help more
while writing/ editing these books.
For my sweet children stepping-up and showing tremendous
kindness by preparing healthy, nutritious
meals because Mommy stayed up through the night
to chronicle adventures.
I am thankful for loving children and such an amazing
husband who has made all this possible with his
tremendous love and support.
2014*

www.FosteringNutrition.com

Contents

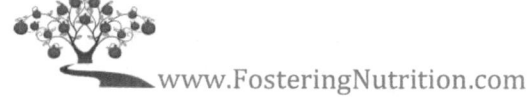
www.FosteringNutrition.com

In Honor of My Parents

Aaron and Seamelia

For showing me how to be generous

Preface

Life is truly amazing. There are good and bad circumstances everyday- and the way we react to these events will shape our children and us.

For a few years, I have remained silent and pondered the purpose of a tragedy. Now I am ready to talk and share; don't worry, I'll share in a positive and hopefully enlightening perspective. Our inspiration is the most precious little foster son. He changed our lives more completely than we realized at the time.

It is also important to note that in this crazy 2 year time span, we are blessed to have the support of my parents and sister as well as special friends, Violet and Juan. There are many friends, but these most notably listened and loved us through this time, where many couldn't handle the injustice. For their kindness, we are truly thankful!

As a mommy, I struggle to inspire my children everyday. I ask….Do I help them become their very best? Do I love them for who they are created to be? My report card comes when my children become young adults and adults. An A+ is that all our children are happy, capable, strong, and so filled with love that they have tremendous ability to love others.

Sometimes, something so incredibly difficult and beautiful happens that it cannot be kept in a box. It

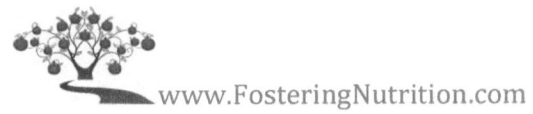 www.FosteringNutrition.com

just takes a little time to understand how to open the box. This was the experience with our family, and my adventure with our very first foster son, then a girl, then sisters, etc... We love each of these children as if our own. And it takes maybe a day to fall in love with a child. The same love as our birth children. Every child is precious and we get so much joy from what each one brings. And with all the good memories, I would be remiss if the really tough memories are not acknowledged. Both make a life worthwhile.

The most shameful memory is desperately wanting to "return a foster child" a few times, because I can, but I don't because my soul won't let me. This is only a taste of an unparalleled journey our family lived out, that collided two worlds together: Fostering and Nutrition. Let me qualify "nutrition": real nutrient-dense, unmodified, food nutrition.

During this unprecedented time we actually have some amazingly fun days. There are some incredibly funny circumstances and of course, the horrific. But this experience is shared because what we encounter impacts everyone, so we attempt to inspire and make a difference in others.

We are the human race and need to start acting like it with the food we eat, the help we give others, and the treatment we administer to the sick.

And a little sappy...as I pray each day and evening for my children, God has given, it is our Nana who started a tradition a few years back. A tradition that we

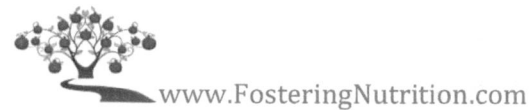

www.FosteringNutrition.com

keep (almost daily) of looking into the sky and noticing what God painted. So when we goof-up, a whole new day awaits us, and God WILL paint a new picture!

So look up. And please enjoy this mini-book that has come at a great cost to our family.

Introduction

When I was a girl of 12 years old, I knew that I wanted to adopt.

Therefore, once I married, my husband and I sought to adopt. We found adoption to be a challenge. You can read more about this in soon-to-be published books by Mandy Lee and Fostering Nutrition.

We decide to help out children that are not able to live at home, and hopefully adopt and provide a permanent home when needed. These children are called foster children in the United States and there are between 460,000 and 500,000 in this system. These children live in orphanage homes or foster family homes.

We are parents committed to our task and in a very short time, we are educated, certified, investigated throughout state and federal databases, cleared, home-inspected, licensed and ready! Incredibly, we receive a child the very same day we are approved to foster.

Our first foster son is 2 years old; adorable, and has been in approximately 4 different homes (could be more) before coming to us. Funny thing is I really

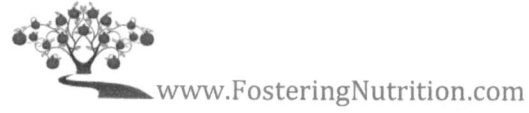

www.FosteringNutrition.com

wanted a girl! I had boys already and needed a little help in the estrogen department; the balance was heavy the other way. Nonetheless, boys are truly wonderful. I certainly love our boys and this new boy comes in and desperately needs to be loved.

After a lot of love, which includes giving parameters, our first foster son is much better prepared for life after only 3 months. Unfortunately, we discover cancer and in two years timing…to the very month of June, we battle cancer, share parenthood, lead health committee decision-making, manage the foster system challenges, endure death and a funeral and try to live on afterward!

As survivors, the lessons we learn are hard ones. It seems criminal and deeply wrong NOT to share and allow others the privilege of learning the easy way. We hope to share our insights with every Parent that we can, in hopes that through our experience you can do better. We hope to; inspire, share existence of options for cancer, and somehow, just maybe a few of you will choose to reach out and help a child.

Please recognize the privilege you have been given to live and grow. May you Blume [or bloom] and grow healthy, live fully, breathe deeply, and be contagious!

We have decided to offer this eBook as a prequel to the more amazing story of Sacrificing the Child that will be published soon.

As I re-live these two years, I will write in the present tense because it is "felt" this way.

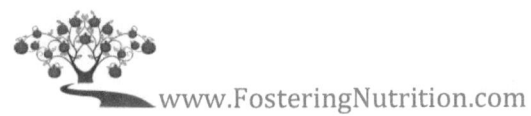
www.FosteringNutrition.com

Our hope is to continually give to these children and as always a portion of proceeds will be given to help children that need a home and a family. Currently, we are underway of building a place that will allow orphan children a place to come, meet animals, harvest food, prepare healthy food, and eat. We hope to inspire all children to choose a wholesome way to live and eat.

Fostering Nutrition with love,
Mandy Lee

1. Value Today

Each day is Important. Not what you think. It is ordinary. It passes s.l.o.w.l.y. in the moment, but fast as you look back.

It can be tough, difficult, moody, fat, skinny, easy, good, bad, frustrating, quiet, loud, peaceful, strife-full. It doesn't matter because it is a day and it is important if YOU acknowledge it is important. This day WILL shape tomorrow. Every single detail, every thought, every breath, every experience will affect the next thought, breath, experience and so on…

Take a deep breath and acknowledge this and then you are ready for:

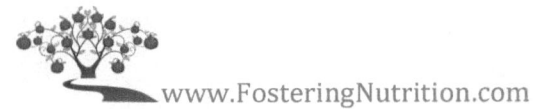
www.FosteringNutrition.com

2. You Are and You Can!

You are exactly who You are supposed to be. Somehow there are moments in life where I spiral down and say the "should've, would've, could've" lines. You know…Oh, if I would've paid attention or planned better, I would be prepared for this situation. Or, I should've gone to that class/seminar/event and this bad situation could've been prevented. Well, as I sit on the hospital bed, with the news that our little guy has cancer, I wish so hard I would've known 3 months ago when I got him. I wish I could've done something to make him better. And in this most deep place, I sit alone, reaching out to God, violently pondering.

In this hanging-space of time a very sweet doctor, touched by God Himself, walks through the door, into my flooded eyes and straight into my soul and speaks these words:

"You are exactly who you are supposed to be. You have done everything you needed to do to be here in this situation today. This moment is defined for you."

He walks out of the room and my insides are screaming in recognition of this unwelcomed truth

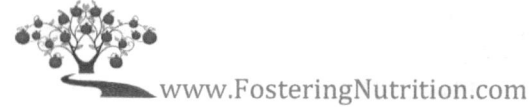

spoken, yet my outside tries not to fall onto the floor and sob so that my precious foster son will have no fear.

Remember this please! Your situation, whether utter devastation or Heavenly surreal-ness, is a part of you. Your experiences have prepared you for these moments. You define who you are in these moments by how you react, but **YOU CAN** handle more than you imagine because **YOU ARE** given each moment based on the hopes and dreams of yesterday.

3. Still…Keep Going

It may get worse! Or it may get incredibly better! These emotions feel similar. Sometimes, when you feel you are at the end of the rope (either in sorrow, despair or elation), you get shown that the rope is longer!

Hang on, don't you dare let go. These are the extraordinary times in life. You may not realize it during the process, but I am certain, these are special times. These are performance times because rehearsal is over! Whatever is in you is oozing out. Go with it to the best of your ability, stay alert, trust your instincts and take note. You will want to evaluate afterwards…but not now.

As a few days pass, I haven't been home to snuggle with my other children. My parents have dropped their lives and come to my home to watch our little guys while I stay at the hospital. My husband works in between visiting all of us. We have not heard from the biological parents and the State is getting worried. Decisions have to be made and the policy in place is to include biological parents if invasive medical needs

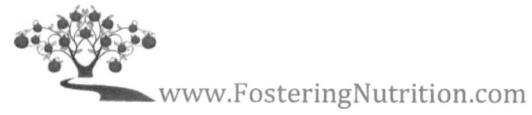

www.FosteringNutrition.com

arise. Well, decisions have been made in our case and neither parent has been reached.

I've lost my diplomacy at this point and begin to order the evaluations and validations for the assessment of our foster son. The State does not know what to do and has too many processes to go through. They can't follow policy because they are unable to reach the parents and the doctors feel trapped with the threat of litigation-whispers filling the unspoken minds. Thus I lose all patience and push action to occur so we can be informed and make decisions, while everyone tells me we have to wait. One doctor comes through. He is able to overcome the fear of litigation with my pressing and assurance of the responsibility to DO what is right. Good grief, right now, I am present and if the courts rule me capable to be his parent, then I will make the decisions! So… we discover, he has cancer…a really nasty, fast moving one. Ugh.

So, just hang on in these times. KEEP GOING; keep moving forward. Afterwards you can look back and assess how you can improve next time. Right now, just be at peace knowing that this too is a learning experience! This is the "in-the-pressure-cooker" moment that actually "shifts" you. You are not alone, even though you feel so. Just Keep Going.

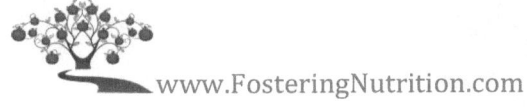

4. ~~CONTROL~~ Overcome Fear

This lesson we all know, but seem to forget until we arrive. **The fear of something is always worse than when "it" arrives.** The anticipation is many times greater than the event. **Balance is everything**. Physiologically your body must balance calcium and magnesium, phosphorous, and other minerals for good bones. Likewise, emotionally we must also balance our caution of a situation and anticipation of what is to come.

For me it is meeting the biological parents. When receiving a child, a file is included that shares the history as it is collected for each foster child… and the amount of information varies. We have medical papers, court rulings on charges against parents, how frequent they get to visit, if they show up, and the family members that try and are unable keep the child. These papers make you cry and over time I learn to skim and avoid somewhat.

Nonetheless, the point is that I am afraid of meeting his biological parents who have drug addictions

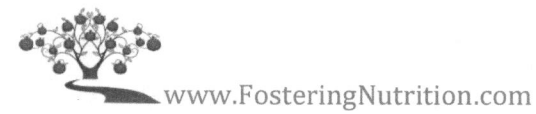

www.FosteringNutrition.com

(prescriptive and non-prescriptive) and domestic violence, as well as prison time.

Before you get too judgmental, you must understand that most of the time their parents were in the "same boat" and did not "hang on" from Chapter 3 and these children grow up and the cycle continues.

Well, I get to meet these people who abandoned/neglected their child, have been in prison, have beat each other…and I am a little nervous.

First, the mom comes in and is devastated. We talk and she catches up on the unfortunate findings. Then the dad comes in and we repeat for him. There are complications with a restraining order for their separation, so my husband and I act as mediators and all is well for a few hours.

It is complicated, but not horrible. In fact, over the next two years, I am privileged to call them my friends. We have been through a lot together…like a dysfunctional family and there is no doubt that I love them.

Whatever your fear, don't try to control it. Rather **Overcome Fear** by just moving through it! Afterwards, you will certainly sigh, but realize this situation <u>has been given to you</u> and you can do this. Even when you don't think you can; you can.

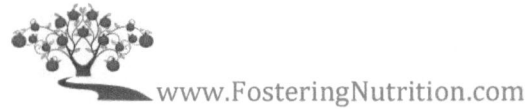

5. Grounding

When **EVERYTHING in your world feels out of your control** and you are doing your best, it is time for grounding. This is a time that you need to sit still for a moment; be quiet. Ponder all that is before you and step back to evaluate. Nothing makes sense, so **FIND YOUR GROUNDING** before you take another action.

It is in this moment that the stream of events hit me. Up until now, I am so busy! I took action to fulfill a dream; it was modified to fostering because of an adoption system that seemed flawed, we went through a rigorous process to be investigated and asked personal questions invading our children's privacy. We have been licensed and brought in a new soul. Now our children have been bruised and bloodied by this child who is lacking real love and my sweet boys are only 4, 5, and 7 years old. We shut down our lives and do not go out in public for two months so we can train and love a child to be a human again. We celebrate improvements and enjoy being a family with 4 boys less than 7 years of age. Then we discover cancer, meet his

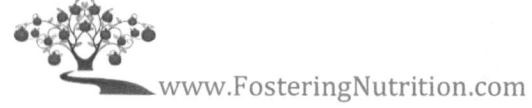

bio-parents whom we must work with, yet still protect our children from their influence. We endure their hatefulness toward each other, their blaming and yelling, sending them out of the hospital, calling the State to let them know our action so it can be legally documented to protect us and the State. And now I sit in my car headed home for the first time after a week.

How in the world am I going to do this? Funny enough, a discussion has already been put to the nine-member committee to get a medical family. We are asked what we think. My husband states how we have invested real time with this child and care about him and believe that God placed him in our care because we are the ones who can handle this. We have genuinely worked to help him be the amazing two-year old boy that is witnessed before them. The Case Manager states that she has known this boy for eight months or so and has never seen him happier and so well mannered. So after a vote (without us in the room), it is agreed that we may continue to keep this child.

Sometimes the "right" thing to do is the "hardest" thing to do. We clearly know this is the right thing to do. So how AM I going to DO this? I homeschool, so the juggling of appointments and hospital time won't be a problem. We can drop everything and do what is needed. We can do school anywhere, with books in tow. So it only comes to the part about the strength. The strength to be around people you don't really

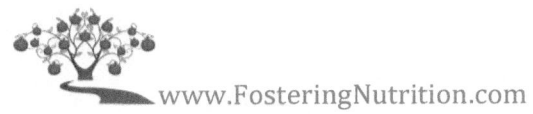

like…**this certainly changes**, but we have been careful whom we allow to influence our children, and we would not choose to be around people like our little guy's biological parents.

I pray. I don't mean, "thank you for this day, please pass the salt," kind-of-prayer. This is the genuine, "You have given this to the wrong person, show me how to do this" prayer. For you it may be different. For me, I have always known there is a Creator of the Universe, within my mind, soul and spirit. It doesn't mean that I haven't ROYALLY screwed up more times than I care to discuss, it just means I know He is there, aware, caring and in control. He let's me choose my life, because FREEDOM of CHOICE is paramount in our nature. So this is my grounding; I pray.

Funny how facing a crisis (whatever it is that devastates you; financial ruin, accident, death, divorce, cancer, etc…) causes clarity! So in this moment of clarity, I pray for us to be all we need to be for Dak and his biological parents and for strength to sustain our marriage and family.

FIND YOUR GROUNDING, pray, and know that time will pass and another season will come and you will be accountable to use what you have been given to **help others**.

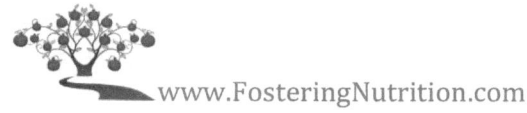

6. Peace Inside

There may NOT be peace all around you, but you can hang on to the peace inside of you.
Very often, **be** reminded to accept the "lot" you have been given. Complaining about your circumstances will not get you out of the circumstances. So find your grounding and resolve to make the best out of it. **Find Peace within**.

I clearly remember the moment we finally come home after a week in the hospital. Arrangements have been made where the bio-parents are able to alternate staying during the nights since the nurses are there to help us supervise. This is a big deal because the State ruled that the bios could not be there unless we were there to supervise and care for our foster son. It was awkward to say the least! So we suggest a "hospital shift" idea and all agree on the 6pm – 9am bio-parent shift and our shift during the day from 9am – 6pm. They need to find jobs and we need to care for our little guy as we were set up to do. The court order is obtained for this arrangement. However, we usually spend an hour or so between shifts talking with each

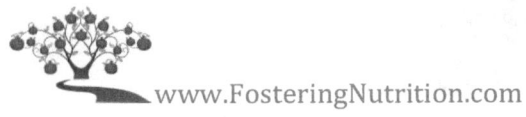

other and downloading the occurrences and findings of the doctors and nurses over the past hours. So, with this court order of our arrangement I get to go home!

I slip in and go to my bathroom decorated in pale blue colors and canvases of Caribbean homes in the water. It is my place of refuge, odd but true. I realize the gravity and begin to cry uncontrollably. My husband respects a bit of time and then he comes in and grabs me by the arms and picks me up. He tells me, "Get a hold of yourself, you have to pull yourself together for the children!" I tell him he is rude (NOT lovingly, of course) and know he is right. I splash cold water on my face in some misguided belief that my puffy, splotchy, red face will look pleasant for the children.

Our children are so precious and standing together as I approach. At such young ages, we hug and begin to cry in a scrunched circle of 4 souls. They ask me if their new brother is going to be ok. At this point, my grounding and source of strength is emboldened as I say, "The Creator of the Universe will allow and do what He will do. We can appeal and pray for His favor, but it does not mean that it will go the way WE think it should go. We must trust and do the very best we can do with each day and love Dak and every person that comes into our path." **There is the peace**. Peace **even** in the parts we don't know, don't like, and certainly do not understand.

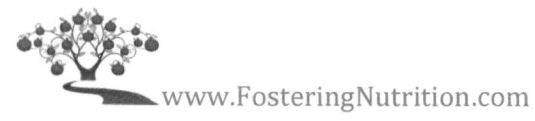 www.FosteringNutrition.com

For when I cry, it is for a reason different than what you are thinking. Not because I don't like this (which is certainly true), but I cry because of the utter horror of it all. When a sweet child is born into this life, abandoned by parents who were not taught and loved well, neglected and alone for gross amounts of time, it is not right. When this same child gets a family willing and able to love and adopt, provide healthy foods, and the child obtains enormous improvement…<u>you just don't get cancer (and age 2)</u>! You've already used up your "bad luck" and now it's the time of "blessing".

Even still, the Master of the Universe is bigger than I understand, so I rest and find peace in Him.

Find your peace, even when it is crazy all around. If I can do it, you certainly can.

7. What you EAT Matters Enormously

What we eat is so important. The deer and wild animals in nature are very precise in what they eat. Sit and observe sometime. Not a domesticated cat or dog, they are lost like us. Eat foods that nourish you. It's an effort each day, and every step is helpful.

Every cell of every tissue that makes up every organ and organ system of our body is made up of what we eat. Food is our fuel just as gasoline is fuel to an automobile. You wouldn't put sludge in your tank if you wanted to drive somewhere, so why put the sludge of refined sugar and refined fat in your body. And then we expect our body to be alert and get up and go somewhere feeling and looking great...**make your food nutrient-dense**.

While in the hospital, canned vitamin milks were given when Dak wouldn't eat. Powdered or chocolate donuts, ice cream, refined bread- the white fluffy stuff. These are not foods you want to give a child, and certainly not a child who is getting an onslaught to every cell in his body through chemotherapy.

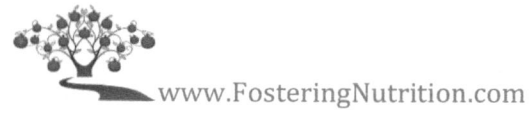 www.FosteringNutrition.com

Physiologically, it doesn't make sense. This is especially the time to be very sensitive with the choice in foods because it is hard to eat, so make it count for good when you finally get hungry.

The funny thing is that I kept teaching Dak to eat healthy and say no to the offerings of bad food. At the same time asking the nurses and biologicals to give him only fresh whole foods. I kept talking about the cells and re-growth. When I went to an amazing school to get certified for Nutritional Therapy, they had the same exact saying about "every cell…" Really, the same exact saying I petitioned the nurses; suffice to say that coincidences are not probable. Merely the Truth is the truth.

If I had a dime for every time a person says, "I eat healthy", I would be wealthy beyond belief. This term is used carelessly in society. From a purest sense, healthy would be to eat real foods that are raw, sometimes cooked, always freshly picked that day, and variety on every plate within available produce of that season. A balance of every protein, carbohydrate, fat, mineral, and vitamin with clean drinking water in the amount needed; all appropriate for your body type and blood type.

This is impossible until the next world! So **get as close as you can. The less items processed, preserved, packaged and shipped in a box or bag, the healthier the food will be.** Stay in the perimeter of the grocery store. Or better yet, find a local

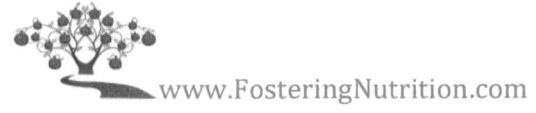

organically-minded farmer in your area. There are Farmer's Markets everywhere. It will help your local economy and feed you more nutrients!

From this it would be really great to affect change in the foods offered to patients in hospitals. Our food is medicine. Somehow we keep forgetting this. Our great-grandparents knew this. They actually ate food. Only since the Industrial Revolution and World Wars did we start packaging and preserving with chemicals. Wouldn't it be fantastic if every hospital would use a **local organic farmer as much as possible**? The hospital could become a place of healing. Almost every doctor I know says to get out as soon as possible because you can't heal in the hospital environment.

So, **eat good, local, nutrient dense food wherever you are**! Your body will be very thankful.

8. Use Your Circumstances to Help Others

For those that have children, "Do you remember how you viewed parents with their children? Did you ever have an idea that you could watch them every second of the day and night, and absolutely nothing would happen to your child?" Well, I mistakenly thought it. And that came flying right back with humility written all over it!

Never think you know all the answers, but use what you have to help others.

Don't view a challenge as a bother; rather realize that you were deemed strong enough to manage it. So **USE IT to affect change** for the positive and **all those after you** will be thankful whether they know you helped them or not.

My family became a spokesperson for health. We help every person that wants it. We teach any person that asks. And we get a lot of opportunities.

I went back to school…again. Learning about nutrition became paramount. My children also learn

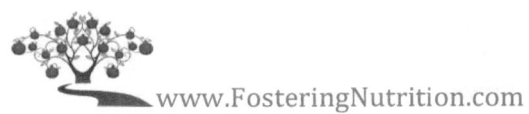

from my schooling. It's a team effort. Hopefully, we all help each other and our community.

We are also a part of a change that occurs in the hospital we've spent so much of our life. A person has been hired specifically to do research and find other successful treatments for pediatric cancer. This hospital now offers alternative treatments for pediatric oncology. We feel a part of this movement as we constantly challenge a better way.

Sharing your knowledge and concerns is a way to change public opinion. We each have experiences that allow growth, inventions, and ideas. The more we share, the greater the chance of eliciting support and when enough people or the right person gets the information, you can change the world for the better.

Unfortunately, **silence** allows public opinion to change without you. Therefore, if you **learn something valuable, make sure you share it**, don't be selfish; **help others.**

So dive in! And **use your situation to help others** that will experience it after you. They will be better for it…and somehow **so will you.**

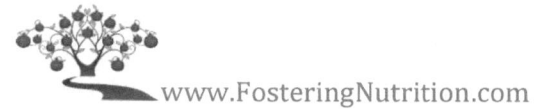

www.FosteringNutrition.com

9. What You SAY Matters Enormously

Oh, the tongue. We can speak blessings or curses; so be very careful with the words you choose to let out of your mouth. Not only will this impact you, but it also affects all those around you. **The power we hold in our tongues is sobering.**

A few years back, I learn of the power of the spoken word, based on Dr. Masaru Emoto's studies. Apparently, Dr. Emoto would speak words to a container of water and then photograph as the water would freeze. He would also write words and tape them to the jar. In his studies, positive words would generate beautiful unique crystals, whereas negative words would crystallize into malformed and ugly crystals. So keep positive, or at least use positive words towards others and since we are approximately 80% water, it surely has a potential to help. Certainly positive words will not harm anyone.

This lesson is one I take up daily. When I am positive and say encouraging words, it seems that the children (and spouse) are all better, happy and behave

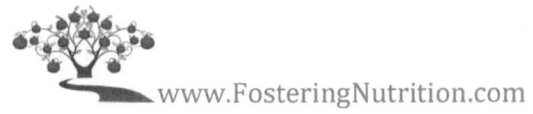

www.FosteringNutrition.com

well. But when I am upset, disappointed and angry, it is a bad day. When I have the self-control to speak life and blessing to my children it matters **significantly**.

We are confined in hospital and clinic rooms for about two years, on and off. It was incredible to experience the power of the tongue. Yes, each of us had bad days. But when we speak kindness to each other, the time in our room passes quickly. These days are amazing. Looking back, it is a miracle how much fun we have. We make a lot of crafts, compare images from our window of what we see painted in the sky, read a lot of great books, learn about each other's favorites, and speak a lot of life into our souls. Fortunately, we have fewer bad days and we continually strive to speak life.

In the last days of Dak's life, he speaks some amazing blessings that we will cherish forever. Even in his tremendous pain, he could still find the power of his little tongue. He asks me to show him the sky. We look quietly out the window with all the children and he whispers, "Look what God painted, Mommy." Then he looks at me and says, "I am ready to be right up there." At four years old, he is tired. I just smile holding back the tears. What power we have with our tongue.

So try this anytime-but here is one of our family-table conversations: At dinner, have each person say one thing nice about a family member. Parents pitch in for the child missed! Also, we find that when correcting a child, it is important to genuinely tell them the amazing things they do and that you are proud of them. Some days it's a hard find, but find something. We all need encouragement. It is astonishing the difference in our family. **Speak blessings using the power of your tongue.**

10. Embrace the Big Moments

Especially embrace the moments you despise in the very core of your being: **embrace!** This is a special chasm of time that will re-define what you believe. If you run from it, you will be scarred for life…and those around you as well. But, **if you embrace the big moments,** many people will be positively moved along with you.

At five o'clock in the morning on a Monday, I get a call from Dak's bio-mom. She is crying and I can hardly understand. She is asking me to come to the hospital quickly, it is really bad this time, our son is flailing around and she cannot do this alone. I barely get the word, "ok" out of my mouth and hang up. I sit and cry and my husband wakes up to ask me what is wrong. As I tell him, he recalls the day before and our activities. It was Sunday, Father's Day, and we had made Father's Day cards; one for bio-Dad and one for Foster Daddy. We had a craft day on Friday with a mess of painting fun. Dak wasn't feeling well at all. It is on this day that he says, "Mommy, I'm ready to go

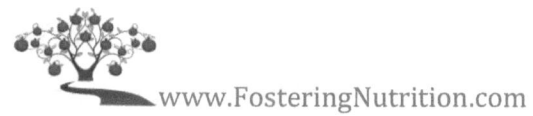

www.FosteringNutrition.com

up there (Heavenward)." On Sunday, we collectively gather and have a Dads' visit; to love this now four-year-old little boy relatively lifeless on the bed.

But now it is Monday at 8am, I am still sitting on the bed gazing at nothing, not wanting to go because it feels bad this time. My friend and Co-mommy is crying and asking for help and I just sat there! Finally, my husband sits down, looks at me and very seriously and calmly with the words, "Embrace this moment." I look at him incredulously and think, "WHAT A JERK!" but say, "what do you mean?" He then relays that this moment began two years ago was given a death sentence by the doctors with a "less than 5%" chance of survival. Now go! And pay attention to the last moments you have.

So, the children and I go to the hospital. As I am halfway there, my friend-nurse calls and tells me I had better hurry! We might not make it. After several awful, near-death experiences, I am genuinely afraid this one is "it" as my foot gets a little heavier on the gas pedal.

We arrive and all our daily security stickers are ready and held by nurse friends and hospital security. We are escorted like VIP into the room and in two hours I have the privilege of holding Dak for the last time and being a part of his spirit moving to the next world (along with his biological Mom and Dad). Only now do I understand the wisdom of my husband and his instructions.

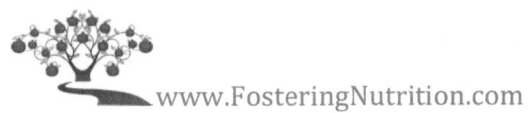

www.FosteringNutrition.com

EMBRACE your big moments, whether good or bad, you will feel your heart and your soul swell within you to truly magnificent heights.

Closing

In closing, I certainly hope my learnings continue as well as yours. Today I stand resolved and growing on many issues regarding health, nutrient-dense food, and training children…but "all-knowing" is not a part of my vernacular. It is —ok NOT to understand everything. It is good to "be loving" instead of hateful. It is gracious to be respectful of those with different opinions. And it is acceptable to NOT have a clue of what-to-do sometimes. These are ways our family chooses to learn and to live; to keep sharing.

There are always options to your treatments and ailments. And although I am not responsible for your health and consulting a doctor is advisable when needed; **YOU are truly responsible for your health**. YOU are empowered to do research when facing anything from a bruised knee to cancer. Know your OPTIONS; don't just blindly go in thinking that the medical system of today is the ONLY way.

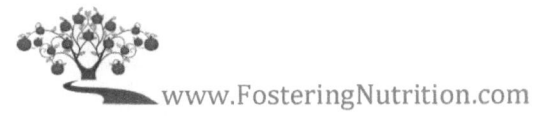

www.FosteringNutrition.com

Here are some cancer treatment options,
http://www.fosteringnutrition.com/cancer-treatments-everyone-know/

1. **Dr.Burzynski Peptide Approach**-Dr. from Poland, discovered success in studies against cancer in 1970s, uses healthy human peptides
2. **Gerson Juice Diet**- practiced in Tijuana, Mexico successfully in a hospital, San Diego, CA for institute in U.S., a plan to juice and starve cancer cells, can do at home
3. **German Freeze Method**- clinics also located in America, treatments for 30 years with systemic treatment usage including hypothermia
4. **Cowan Holistic Approach**-systemic approach from a Natural doctor who has found tremendous success
5. **Dr. Gonzales,** Medical Doctor who evaluates metabolic type and treats systemically with any of these above treatment approaches and more
6. **<u>Essential Oils</u>**- medical research shows heightened potency and many successful studies show Frankincense oil to be effective, from the country of Oman.
7. Chemotherapy, really this one needs no link, you will get this information everywhere.

My refrigerator is my pharmacy. I have medical and holistic friends, as well as personally going to school to become a Nutritional Therapy Practitioner. Be

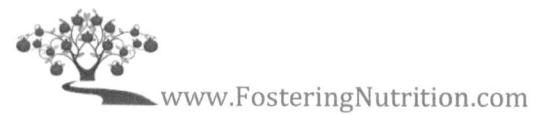

www.FosteringNutrition.com

informed and prepared…we were not, but now we are certainly better prepared. I never dreamed of cancer in a child. Now I know that 1 in 5 children born as of the year 2000 will get cancer. 1 in 3 children will have pediatric diabetes, unless something is drastically changed. Source: Nutritional Therapy Association (http://nutritionaltherapy.com). I believe the answer lies in the food we eat to REDUCE these epidemic levels of disease. There is a whole floor area in most hospitals dedicated to pediatric cancer and it's a growing business. Eye-opening doesn't quite cover our sentiments.

In parting, I wish you the greatest gift of life. May you continue to grow and be the amazing person you are created to be. May you find life's true love and what He paints for you. And then, may you share that love by helping others, forgiving and showing grace as we learn how to live.

Remember to notice the heavenly artwork each day and observe how it emerges into a new beautiful picture. As you find joy in each child, remember tomorrow is a whole new day and a picture you haven't even seen! A day to; love better, eat better, and live better! And may we love all the children; birth, foster, and adopted and therefore create a better tomorrow.

And be sure to check us out as we seek to share our healthy living and continue Fostering Nutrition at: www.fosteringnutrition.com and on Facebook, Pinterest, and Google +.

www.ingramcontent.com/pod-product-compliance
Lightning Source LLC
Chambersburg PA
CBHW050524290526
45786CB00007B/2684